C000133173

C-reactive protein – A diagnostic marker

An Acute Phase Reactant

LAP LAMBERT Academic Publishing

Impressum / Imprint

Bibliografische Information der Deutschen Nationalbibliothek: Die Deutsche Nationalbibliothek verzeichnet diese Publikation in der Deutschen Nationalbibliografie; detaillierte bibliografische Daten sind im Internet über http://dnb.d-nb.de abrufbar.
Alle in diesem Buch genannten Marken und Produktnamen unterliegen warenzeichen-, marken- oder patentrechtlichem Schutz bzw. sind Warenzeichen oder eingetragene Warenzeichen der jeweiligen Inhaber. Die Wiedergabe von Marken, Produktnamen, Gebrauchsnamen, Handelsnamen, Warenbezeichnungen u.s.w. in diesem Werk berechtigt auch ohne besondere Kennzeichnung nicht zu der Annahme, dass solche Namen im Sinne der Warenzeichen- und Markenschutzgesetzgebung als frei zu betrachten wären und daher von jedermann benutzt werden dürften.

Bibliographic information published by the Deutsche Nationalbibliothek: The Deutsche Nationalbibliothek lists this publication in the Deutsche Nationalbibliografie; detailed bibliographic data are available in the Internet at http://dnb.d-nb.de.
Any brand names and product names mentioned in this book are subject to trademark, brand or patent protection and are trademarks or registered trademarks of their respective holders. The use of brand names, product names, common names, trade names, product descriptions etc. even without a particular marking in this works is in no way to be construed to mean that such names may be regarded as unrestricted in respect of trademark and brand protection legislation and could thus be used by anyone.

Coverbild / Cover image: www.ingimage.com

Verlag / Publisher:
LAP LAMBERT Academic Publishing
ist ein Imprint der / is a trademark of
AV Akademikerverlag GmbH & Co. KG
Heinrich-Böcking-Str. 6-8, 66121 Saarbrücken, Deutschland / Germany
Email: info@lap-publishing.com

Herstellung: siehe letzte Seite /
Printed at: see last page
ISBN: 978-3-659-28347-5

Zugl. / Approved by: Bangalore, Rajiv Gandhi University of Health Sciences, Diss., 2005

CONTENTS

INTRODUCTION

C-reactive protein is an acute phase reactant released by the body in response to acute injury or other inflammatory stimuli and is a fundamental response of the body to injury (Tillet and Francis 1930).[1] CRP is a serum protein synthesized in liver only during an inflammatory disease   (Gewurz H., et al 1982)[2] and has a half-life of 19 hrs. It is normally present as a trace constituent of plasma (0 to 0.6mg/dl). CRP concentration increases in the blood in association with inflammation or tissue destruction and the termination of the process is accompanied by a return of the CRP level to normal.[2] The rate of synthesis and secretion increases within hours of an acute injury or onset of inflammation. It may reach as high as 20 times the normal value.[3] It plays a protective role in recognizing foreign pathogens and initiating their elimination, probably activating the classic pathway of complement through C-activation.[4]

An elevated serum concentration of CRP is an evidence of active tissue–damaging process[1] and CRP is an indicator of current disease activity. Numerous studies have been conducted comparing the CRP levels in assessing the disease activity of various systemic inflammatory disorders and in diagnosing and management of systemic infections.

Raised CRP levels have been observed in conditions like rheumatoid arthritis, ankylosing spondilitis, wegener's granulomatosis, polyarteritis nodosa, Behcet's syndrome, neonatal septicemia, systemic lupus erythematosus, post operative infection, thromboembolic complications after major surgery, ulcerative colitis, myocardial infarction.[1]

Recent studies have shown that C-Reactive protein serum levels in patients with periodontal disease are elevated. Periodontal pathogens affect local and systemic immune and inflammatory responses. The local inflammatory response to those gram-bacteria or bacterial products is characterized by infiltration of the periodontal tissues of inflammatory cells, including polymorphonuclear neutrophils (PMN), macrophages, lymphocytes, and plasma cells. Activated macrophages release cytokines, and some individuals respond to microbial challenge with an abnormally high delivery of such inflammatory mediators such as PGE_2, IL-1 and 6and TNF-α. These cytokines are involved in destruction of both periodontal connective tissue and alveolar bone.[5]

There is increasing evidence that chronic infections as well as inflammatory mechanisms play a major role in atherogenesis and cardiovascular diseases (CVD). Several studies suggested an association between periodontal diseases and atherosclerosis. Direct and indirect host-mediated effects of infectious agents may be responsible for the association between infections in general and periodontitis specifically, and atherosclerosis.[5]

Recent investigations suggested that even a moderate increase in CRP levels, such as those found in periodontitis patients, may predict a risk for atherosclerosis and cardiovascular diseases. The mechanism by which CRP participates in cardiovascular diseases is not clear; however, CRP may activate the complement system and be involved in foam cell formation in atheromas.[5]

REVIEW OF
LITERATURE

GENERAL REVIEW :

Historical Introduction :

The discovery of C-Reactive Protein (CRP) was reported in 1930 by Tillet and Francis.[1] They were investigating serological reactions in pneumonia with various extracts of pneumococci and observed that a non-specific somatic polysaccharide fraction, which they designated fraction C, was precipitated by the sera of acutely ill patients. After the crisis the capacity of the patient's sera to precipitate C polysaccharide (CPS) rapidly disappeared, and the C-reactive material was not found in sera from normal healthy individuals.

Avery (1941)[1] and his collaborators characterized the C-reactive material as a protein which required calcium ions for its reaction with CPS (C-polysaccharide) and introduced the term "acute phase" to refer to serum from patients acutely ill with infectious disease and containing the C-reactive protein.

Lofstrom (1944)[1] independently described a non-specific capsular-swelling reaction of some strains of pneumococci when mixed with acute-phase sera and subsequently showed that the substance responsible was CRP. He detected CRP in non-infectious as well as infectious conditions; and the acute – phase reaction, in which the concentration of certain plasma proteins increases, is now recognized as a general and non-specific response to most forms of infective and non-infective inflammatory processes, cellular and / or tissue necrosis, and malignant neoplasia semi-quantitative assays for serum CRP were widely used for many years to provide an objective index of the acute-phase response and therefore of disease activity

6

in rheumatological and other conditions. The dramatic changes in CRP concentration which occur in disease suggest that it may have important physiological and / or pathophysiological functions.

Synthesis, Structure And Binding Properties Of CRP:

CRP is synthesized by hepatocytes and is normally present as a trace constituent of the plasma. The rate of CRP synthesis and secretion increases within hours of an acute injury or the onset of inflammation, probably under the influence of humoral mediators, such as leucocyte endogenous mediator (endogenous pyrogen) and prostaglandin PGE_1. The serum CRP concentration may reach peak levels of as much as 300 µg/ml within 24-48 hours.[1]

Human CRP is found in plasma as a non-glycosylated cyclic pentamer consisting of identical 21,000 dalton non-covalently bound subunits. In primates and rabbits the concentration of CRP in plasma increases 100 to 1000 fold after tissue injury or inflammation. This increase in CRP concentration exceeds by several orders of magnitude the increase noted for other acute phase serum proteins, such as haptoglobin, fibrinogen, α_1-antitrypsin, α_1-antichymotrypsin, α_1-acid glycoprotein, C_3 (the third complement (C) component), and ceruloplasmin. Only the increase in serum amyloid A protein (SAA), after tissue injury is comparable to that for CRP.[6]

Immunohistochemical examination of rabbit liver and biosynthetic studies of primary tissue cultures indicate that liver is the major, if not only, site of CRP synthesis. The in vivo rate of catabolism of radiolabeled CRP is rapid and not significantly different in normal animals and in animals stimulated with endotoxin or turpentine, supporting the conclusion that the acute phase increase

7

in serum CRP is due to an increased rate of synthesis. Induction of CRP synthesis may be mediated by blood-borne factors, similar or identical with IL-1, a product of mononuclear phagocytes that induces SAA synthesis.[6]

For several reasons, the induction of CRP synthesis after tissue injury serves as an excellent model for studies of eukaryotic gene control.[6]

a) The increase in CRP synthesis is quantitatively impressive i.e., the CRP levels in human plasma under "resting" conditions is about 1to 2µg/ml. Within hours after tissue injury, plasma levels exceeding 100 µg/ml are observed.

b) The protein has been purified to homogeneity; its complete amino acid sequence is known and some of its biologic activities have been elucidated.

c) Analogous proteins are found in many species including rather primitive invertebrates, such as Limulus polyphemus (horse shoe crab) in which the protein is a constitutive product. In the Syrian hamster, production of the analogous protein is apparently under the control of sex hormones as well as mediators of the acute phase response.

d) CRP cDNA clones have been isolated and are available for studies of the structure and expression of the CRP gene.[6]

Structural Biology And Host Defence Function :

Czalai A.J., et al (1999)[7] described human CRP as a calcium (Ca^{2+}) binding acute phase protein with binding specificity for phosphocholine. Recent crystallographic and mutagenesis studies have provided a solid understanding of the structural biology of the protein; while experiments using transgenic mice have confirmed its host defense function. The protein consists of five identical protomers each containing 187 amino acids, with one intrachain disulfide bond and no carbohydrate modification in a disc-like configuration in a cyclic symmetry. On one face of each protomer there is a binding site for phosphocholine consisting of two Ca^{2+} ions that ligate the phosphate group and a hydrophobic pocket that accommodates the methyl groups of phosphocholine. On the opposite face is a deep cleft formed by parts of the N and C termini and bordered by an alpha–helix. Mutational studies indicate that the $C1_Q$-binding site of the molecule is located at the open end of this cleft with Asp 112 and Tyr 175 representing contact residues. Using human CRP transgenic mice, Czalai et al (1999) investigated the host – defense functions of the protein. Transgenic mice infected with streptococcus pneumonia had increased lifespan and lowered mortality compared to wild-type mice. This was attributable to an upto 400 fold reduction in bacteremia mediated mainly by the interaction of CRP with complement.

The Physiologic Structure Of Human CRP and its Complex With Phosphocholine :

Human CRP is the classical acute phase reactant, the circulating concentration of which rises rapidly and extensively in a cytokine-mediated response to tissue injury, infection and inflammation, serum CRP values are routinely measured, empirically, to detect and monitor human diseases (Thompson D., Pepys M.B. and Wood S.P. 1999) However, CRP is likely to have important host defense, scavenging and metabolic functions through its capacity for calcium dependent binding to exogenous and autologous molecules

9

containing phosphocholine (PC) and then activating the classical complement pathway. CRP may also have pathogenic effects and the recent discovery of a prognostic association between increased CRP production and coronary atherothrombotic events is of particular interest.[8]

The X-ray structures of fully calcified, CRP, in the presence and absence of bound PC, reveal that although the subunit beta-sheet jellyroll fold is very similar to that of the homologous pentameric protein serum amyloid P component, each subunit is tipped towards the fivefold axis. PC is found in a shallow surface pocket on each subunit, interacting with the two protein-bound calcium ions via the phosphate group and with glu 8 / via the choline moiety. There is also an unexpected hyprobic pocket adjacent to the ligand.[8]

The structure shows how large ligands containing PC may be bound by CRP via a phosphate oxygen that projects away from the surface of the protein. Multipoint attachment of one palmar face of the CRP molecule to a PC bearing surface would leave available, on the opposite exposed face, the recognition sites for C1q, which have been identified by mutagenesis. This would enable CRP to target physiologically and/or pathologically significant complement activation. The hydrophobic pocket adjacent to bound PC invites the design of inhibitors of CRP binding, that may have therapeutic relevance to the possible role and CRP in atherothrombotic events.[8]

Proteins Related To C-Reactive Protein And Synthesis :

The acute phase proteins have been found to have an essential role in the inhibition of extracellular proteases, blood clotting, fibrinolysis, modulation of immune cell function and the neutralization and clearance of harmful components from the circulation.[9]

The synthesis of these acute phase proteins has been shown to be regulated by cytokines and to a lesser extent by glucocorticoid hormones. The majority of the acute-phase proteins are glycoproteins, which play a variety of roles in the homeostatic response to injury. The acute phase proteins in humans differ-substantially in the magnitude of their rise after onset of injury. The serum concentration of a number of those proteins increases rapidly during infection and concentrations can increase 2 to 100 fold and remain elevated throughout infection[9].

Acute phase proteins can be divided into two groups: Type I and Type II [9]

Type I : Proteins include serum amyloid A, C-reactive protein, complement C_3 and α_1-acid glycoprotein, which are induced by the proinflammatory, IL-1 like cytokines (IL-1 and tumor necrosis factor).

Type II : Proteins include fibrinogen, haptoglobin, α_1-antichymotrypsin, α_1-antitrypsin, α_2-macroglobulin and are induced by the IL-6 like cytokines.[9]

The α-helical cytokines; IL-6 and oncostatin M, are the most potent recognized inducers of acute phase proteins. The effect of IL-6 on the production of hepatic proteins can also be influenced significantly by other cytokines and by insulin and the counter regulatory hormones (dexamethasone, glucagon, and epinephrine). In general, IL-6 like cytokines synergize with IL-1 like cytokines to induce type I acute phase proteins. This phenomenon is thought to

11

be principally controlled by IL-6 acting on the hepatocyte and inducing transcriptional activation of the acute-phase protein genes. As such, type I acute phase protein genes contain nuclear factor-kB, nuclear factor IL-6 and AP-1 response elements in their promoter regions, whereas type II acute phase protein genes contain a hexanulceotide motif (CTGGGA), which is an IL-6 response element.[9]

The reciprocal interaction between IL-6 and functionally related other inflammatory cytokines, as well as the hypothalamo-pituitary adrenal axis, represents a separate fact of the complex web of regulatory neuroendocrino immunological interactions. Glucocorticosteroids decrease the level of IL-1, tumor necrosis factor and IL-6 in the peripheral blood via transcriptional and post-transcriptional routes and prolong their impact on the target cells through the elevation of the expression of their receptors. While endogenous pyrogen (IL-1) is well known to cause fever, IL-6 can also induce fever. Finally, there exist apparent feedback mechanisms involving both liver synthesized acute-phase proteins and neuroendocrine factors from the central nervous system, which contribute to regulation of the acute phase response to inflammation.[9]

Serum amyloid P (SAP), a normal human plasma protein (mean $\pm$ SD normal concentration 37 $\pm$ 12 μg / ml) is closely related to CRP and resembles it structurally and in having calcium dependent ligand binding capacity. This latter property was first discovered with respect to agarose, and serum proteins which undergo calcium dependent binding to agarose have been isolated

12

form elasmobranches, teleost fish and amphibia, as well as mammals. They all closely resemble human SAP in molecular appearance, and plaice SAP- the only one to have been partly sequenced shows about 50% homology with human SAP. CRP and SAP thus form a distinct family of plasma proteins, with unique molecular configuration, amino acid sequence, and specific calcium dependent ligand binding capacity, which have been stably conserved throughout vertebrate evolution.[1]

Functional Properties Of C-Reactive Protein :

CRP precipitates soluble ligands and agglutinates particulate ligands. Once complexed, via either its calcium dependent or its polycation binding sites, it becomes a potent activator of the classical complement pathway starting with C1q. Complement activation proceeds as efficiently as with an IgG antibody and leads to fixation of C_{4b} and C_{3b}, which can mediate the important complement dependent adherence reactions, and to fixation of the terminal complex C_{5b}-C_9, causing lysis if the ligand is on a cell surface. Complement split fragments, active in the fluid phase, are also generated. CRP, like antibodies, can thus bind to ligands, opsonise materials for phagocytosis, and initiate cell-damaging and inflammatory reactions.[1]

Other activities which have been ascribed to CRP include selective binding to T-lymphocytes and modification of some of their functions, suppression of platelet aggregation and activation reactions, and enhancement of the activity and motility of phagocytic cells. CRP complexed in a suitable way may bind to lymphocytes bearing Fc(γ) receptors (including B, T and non-B, non-T cells) both in vivo and in vitro, but the functional significance of this is not known.[1]

Regulation Of Complement Activation By CRP :

Mold C., Gewurz H. and Du-Clos T.W. (1999)[10] stated CRP as an acute phase serum protein and a mediator of innate immunity. CRP binds to microbial polysaccharides and to ligands exposed on damaged cells. Binding of CRP to those substrates activates the classical complement pathway leading to their uptake by phagocytic cells. Complement activation by CRP is restricted to C_1, C_4 and C_3 with little consumption of C_{5-9}. Surface bound CRP reduces deposition and generation of C_{5b-9} by the alternative pathway and depositions of C_{3b} and lysis by the lectin pathway. These activities of CRP are the result of recruitment of factor H resulting in regulation of C_{3b} on bacteria or erythrocytes. Evidence is presented for direct binding of H to CRP. H binding to CRP or C_{3b} immobilized on microtiter wells was demonstrated by ELISA. Attachment of CRP to a surface was required for H binding. H binding to CRP was not inhibited by EDTA or phosphocholine, which inhibit ligand binding, but was inhibited by a 13 amino acid CRP peptide. The peptide sequence was identical to the region of CRP that showed the best alignment to H binding peptides from streptococcus pyogenes (M6) and Neisseria gonorrhoeae (Pocl A). The results suggest that CRP bound to a surface provides secondary binding sites for H resulting in greater regulation of alternative pathway amplification and C_5-convertases. Complement activation by CRP may help limit the inflammatory response by providing opsonization with minimal generation of C_{5a} and C_{5b-9}.[10]

Regulation Of Phagocytic Leucocyte Activities By CRP :

Mortensen R.F. and Zhong W. (2000)[11] classified the classic acute phase reactant CRP as an effector of innate host resistance because it activates the classical complement cascade and is opsonic. The latter occurs via specific CRP receptors (CRP-R) that have recently been identified as both Fc gamma RI and Fc gamma RII on human phagocytic leucocytes. New findings also suggest an anti-inflammatory role for CRP because it modulates endotoxin shock and inhibits chemotaxis and the respiratory burst of neutrophils. CRP inhibited phorbol myristate acetate-induced superoxide (O_2) production more efficiently than the fMLP-triggered response. An examination of the inhibition of the proteins kinase C (PKC) – dependent assembly of the NADPH oxidase complex revealed that both phosphorylation and translocation of PKC-beta 2 to the membrane were inhibited by a threshold acute phase dose of approximately 50 μg / ml CRP. Translocation of the membrane and serine-phosphorylation of the major cytosolic p47-phox component of the NADPH oxidase complex was inhibited by CRP. CRP also inhibited membrane localization of activated Rac2, the small G protein regulator of the assembly of the oxidase components in activated neutrophils as well as the cytoskeleton during chemotactic movement. CRP-mediated regulation occurs via the CRP-R because an IgM mouse mAb to the human CRP-P mimicked CRP may serve as an anti-inflammatory regulator of activities at sites of tissue damage where it selectively accumulates and thus influences neutrophil infiltration and polymorphonuclear neutrophil activities. By contrast, CRP activates cells of the monocyte / macrophage lineage, suggesting differential regulation of these two leucocyte populations at the level of signalling. CRP appears to be a multifunctional protein with the capability of exerting both effector functions for innate host resistance, as well as existing specific anti-inflammatory effects.[11]

Effects Of CRP On Human Lymphocyte Responsiveness :

Vitter M.L., et al (1982)[12] stated CRP, as a trace serum protein shown to bind to a subset of human IgG-FcR-bearing peripheral blood lymphocytes (PBL) in the presence of a ligand such as pneumococcal C-polysaccharide (CPS). CRP has also been detected on a small percentage of PBL that are associated with NK activity. In the present study, they assessed the effects of CRP and CRP-CPS complexes on a variety of human lymphocyte functions in vitro CRP and CRP complexes significantly enhanced (generally 2 to 3 fold) cell-mediated cytotoxicity, minimally enhanced the MLC (mixed lymphocyte culture) reaction and induced a small but regularly detectable blastogenic response in resting PBL. CRP or CRP-CPS complexes had no effect on nitrogen induced blastogenesis; PWM (poke weed mitogen) induced generation of IgM plaque-forming cells; E rosette formation, Ab-dependent cell-mediated cytotoxicity or NK-activity.[12]

The Role of C-Reactive Protein In Vivo : A Hypothesis

The role of CRP in vivo is not known, although under some circumstances it can cause inflammation. CRP may play a part in the pathogenesis of the many inflammatory conditions in which its circulating concentration is elevated. Probably the normal function of CRP is generally beneficial to the organism as a whole, and this may be by acting as an early broad-spectrum recognition mechanism for the products of pathogenic microorganisms. On the other hand increased CRP production is a feature of non-infective as well as infective diseases, and CRP binds to a wide range of autogenous products– lipids and phospholipids, polycations and polyanions – all of which are constituents of cells and likely to be abnormally exposed in or released from damaged tissues. In vivo-binding of CRP to necrotic cells has been described and may contribute to resolution and repair. The main role of CRP is to recognize in the plasma the potentially toxic autogenous materials released from damaged tissues, to bind to them, and thereby to detoxify them and / or facilitate their clearance.[1]

Measurement Of Serum C-Reactive Protein In Clinical Practice :

Measurement of serum CRP is useful in the following clinical settings: [1]

1) Screening test for organic disease:
   - Outpatient consultation
   - 'Well' person screening

2) Assessment of disease activity in inflammatory disorders :
   - Rheumatoid arthritis
   - Juvenile chronic arthritis
   - Ankylosing spondylitis
   - Reiter's syndrome
   - Psoriatric arthropathy
   - Vasculitic syndromes (polymyalgia rheumatica, Wegener's granulomatosis, polyarteritis nodosa, Behcet's syndrome)
   - Crohn's disease.
   - Rheumatic fever
   - Familial Mediterranean fever.

3) Diagnosis and Management of infection :
- Neonatal septicaemia and meningitis
- Intercurrent infection in systemic lupus erythematosus
- Intercurrent infection in leukaemia
- Post operative infection (and thromboembolic complications after major surgery)

4) Differential diagnosis / classification of inflammatory disorders :
- Systemic lupus erythematosus versus rheumatoid arthritis and other arthritides.
- Crohn's disease versus ulcerative colitis.

5) Miscellaneous :
- Assessment of myocardial infarction

An elevated serum concentration of CRP is unequivocal evidence of an active tissue damaging process, and CRP measurement thus provides a simple screening test for organic disease.[1]

CRP AND PERIODONTITIS

The pathogenetic role of the subgingival microbiota in the initiation and progression of periodontitis is widely accepted. Periodontal pathogens affect local and systemic immune and inflammatory responses. The local inflammatory response to these gram bacteria or bacterial products is characterized by infiltration of the periodontal tissues of inflammatory cells including polymorphonuclear neutrophils (PMN), macrophages, lymphocytes, and plasma cells. Activated macrophages release cytokines, and some individuals respond to microbial challenge with an abnormally high delivery of such inflammatory mediators as PGE_2, IL-1 and TNF-α.[5]

These cytokines are involved in destruction of both periodontal connective tissue and alveolar bone. They can also initiate a systemic acute phase response. Recent studies have shown that C-reactive proteins (CRP) serum levels in patients with periodontal disease are elevated.[5]

Craig R.G., et al (2003)[13] conducted a study to determine the effect of destructive periodontal disease, status, severity and progression on components of the acute phase response in an urban minority population. They assessed probing depth, attachment level, gingival erythema, bleeding upon probing, suppuration and plaque. CRP was measured using a high sensitivity CRP (hsCRP) assay. They suggested that destructive periodontal disease and disease progression are associated with changes in serum components consistent with an acute phase response.

19

Ide M., et al (2003)[14] conducted a study to ascertain if circulating levels of cardiovascular and systemic inflammatory markers could be modified following treatment of periodontal disease. Periodontal examination including probing depth, loss of attachment, plaque scores and bleeding scores were assessed in adult subjects. Venous blood was analysed to determine serum and plasma fibrinogen, C-reactive protein, sialic acid, tumour necrosis factors α and IL-6, and 1β. They reported that improvement in periodontal health did not influence the levels of vascular markers.

Noack B., et al (2001)[5] conducted a study to examine whether CRP plasma levels are increased in periodontitis and if there is a relation to severity of periodontal disease and to the periodontal microflora. CRP levels were assessed using radial immunodiffusion assay. The presence of periodontal pathogens Pg, Pi, Cr, Bf (Porphyromonas Gingivalis, Prevotella Intermedia, Campylobacter Rectus, Bacteroides Forsythus) in the subgingival plaque samples was measured by immunofluorescence microscopy. It was concluded that the extent of increase in CRP levels in periodontitis patients depends on the severity of the disease after adjusting for age, smoking, body mass-index, triglycerides and cholesterol.

Mario, et al (2001)[15] investigated the CRP pattern production after stroke and whether different pattern were associated with outcomes in 193 patients with first ever ischemic stroke. They stated that CRP is a sensitive marker of inflammation and its level identify those patients whose inflammation system responds most actively to stimuli and the inflammatory reaction caused by an ischemic stroke is measurable by determination of CRP concentration, the levels of which predicts the outcome. They concluded that periodontal disease and CRP could be useful markers because they can identify a group of patients at higher risk.

Wu T., et al (2000)[16] conducted a study to examine the relation between periodontal health and cardiovascular risk factors: serum total and high density lipoproteins cholesterol, C-Reactive protein and plasma fibrinogen. The results of their study indicated a significant relation between indicators of poor periodontal status and increased CRP and fibrinogen. They found a weak association between periodontal status and total cholesterol level, while no consistent association between periodontal status and high density lipoprotein cholesterol. They concluded that total choldesterol, CRP and fibrinogen are possible intermediate factors that may link periodontal disease to elevated cardiovascular risk.

Ebersole J.L. and Cappelli D. (2000)[9] reported that CRP promotes the binding of complement, when bound to bacteria and facilitates their uptake by phagocytes. They also reported that CRP did not appear to be a typical antibody to pneumococcus for several reasons i) CRP is present in sera from patients with other bacterial illness. ii) CRP is not detectable in the sera from normal individuals; and iii) the concentration of CRP rapidly decreases in patients who recovered from pneumonia, whereas typical antibody responses are generally elevated in convalescence. CRP is normally present in ng/ml quantities but may increase dramatically to hundred of μg/ml within 72 hours following tissue injury. They reported that measurement of serum CRP can provide a valuable and timely barometer for many disease processes, including infections, as well as non-infectious conditions. CRP reacts with cell surface receptors, resulting in opsonization, enhanced phagocytosis and passive protection; activation of the classical complement pathway; scavenger for chromatin fragments; inhibition of growth and / or metastasis of tumor cells; and modulation of polymorphonuclear leucocytes function.

Williams R.C., and Offenbacher S. (2000)[17] reported that periodontitis is significantly associated with several conditions, including myocardial infarction, stroke and preterm delivery. They reported that periodontitis can elicit a systemic inflammatory response by activating the hepatic acute phase response as a consequence of transient and recurrent bacteremia of oral origin. They also reported that periodontitis elicits a mild elevation in markers of acute phase response, including CRP, haptoglobin, α1-antitrypsin and fibrinogen. The acute phase response is triggered by blood-borne oral lipopolysaccharide and oral bacteria which elicit the release of the cytokines interleukin-6 and tumor necrosis factor-α. These mediators act in the liver to induce the acute phase response and hepatic secretion of these serum acute-phase proteins. They hypothesized that measures of periodontal infection should be considered as one of the potential underlying causes of both increased levels of acute-phase response proteins and the attendant increase in cardiovascular risk.

Loos B.G., et al (2000)[18] conducted a study to evaluate the systemic markers related to cardiovascular diseases in the peripheral blood of periodontitis patients. They assessed the IL-6 and CRP levels and leucocyte counts in patients with generalized and localized

22

periodontitis and compared the results with healthy controls. They concluded that periodontitis results in higher systemic levels of CRP, IL-6 and neutrophils and reported that these elevated inflammatory factors may increase inflammatory activity in atherosclerotic lesions, potentially increasing the risk for cardiac or cerebrovascular events.

Slade G.D., et al (2000)[19] conducted a study to evaluate associations among periodontal disease, established risk factors for elevated CRP and CRP levels within the US population and to determine whether total loss is associated with reduced CRP. CRP was quantified from peripheral blood samples and analyzed as a continuous variable and as the prevalence of elevated CRP ($\geq$10 mg/L). It was found that dentate people with extensive periodontal disease had an increase of approximately 1/3 in mean CRP and a doubling in prevalence of elevated CRP compared with periodontally healthy people. Raised CRP levels with extensive periodontal disease persisted in multivariate analysis with established risk factors for elevated CRP (diabetes, arthritis, emphysema, smoking and anti-inflammatory medications) and sociodemographic factors controlled for.

Ebersole J.L., et al (1999)[20] conducted a study to investigate the general mechanisms which could describe the association of systemic diseases processes, including i) systemic translocation of bacteria / products during periodontitis ii) Alterations in systemic inflammatory biomarkers during periodontitis iii) the relationship of periodontitis to serum lipids / lipoproteins. The serum levels of various acute phase reactants and chemokines. (eg. CRP, α_1-antitrypsin, haptoglobin, fibrinogen,IL-8) was determined. They observed specific changes in serum lipid levels (cholesterol, triglycerides, HDL, LDL) and lipoproteins (apo A-1) during periodontitis in non-human primates. They thus concluded that systemic manifestations of periodontitis that include detection of bacterial products, inflammatory biomarkers and dyslipoproteinemia consistent with and increased atherogenic risk.

Frederiksson M.I., et al (1999)2[1] conducted a study to compare the systemic effects of periodontitis and cigarette smoking separately and in combination, in order to study the hyper-reactivity in peripheral neutrophils. Blood cells and acute-phase proteins were studied. The generation of free oxygen radicals from neutrophils was measured as luminol enhanced chemiluminescence (CL) after activation of their Fc_γ receptors with opsonized staphylococcus aureus. They concluded that the effects of periodontitis on CRP and IgG_2 means that periodontal lesions may also leak agents, priming the peripheral neutrophils to increased chemiluminescence (CL).

Glurich I., et al (1998)[22] conducted a study to assess if inflammation associated with periodontal disease could contribute to atherogenesis. Sera from subjects whose periodontal disease and cardiovascular status were known, were tested by ELISA for levels of CRP, SAA, phospholipase A_2 (SPLA$_2$) and interleukin 1β and 6, proinflammatory cytokines associated with acute phase regulation. It was concluded that the host response to periodontal disease and cardiovascular disease is reflected by increased acute phase protein levels and subjects with both periodontal disease and cardiovascular disease exhibited higher levels of SAA and CRP than those with one

24

or controls with neither condition, suggesting a role for these acute phase proteins.

Ebersole J.L., et al (1997)[23] conducted a study to determine the relationship between periodontal status and both CRP and haptoglobin levels at baseline, to follow the CRP and haptoglobin levels over time and to assess any changes in CRP and haptoglobin subsequent to both local and then systemic periodontal therapy. They found that CRP and haptoglobin were significantly elevated in patients with the most disease active sites over a 6 month period. CRP levels declined by 35-40% after 1-2 year of treatment with the drug (Flurbiprofen). They concluded that either these molecules are formed locally and distributed to the serum, or these presumably localized infections impact upon the systemic components of the host protective responses.

Meurman J.H., et al (1997)[24] investigated 191 elderly patients referred to an acute geriatric hospital due to sudden worsening of their general health in the age group of 67 to 96 years. Medical examination and erythrocyte sedimentation rates (ESR) and serum C-reactive protein concentrations were analyzed during the first day in the hospital. They concluded that high ESR and CRP values were observed in connection with infectious diseases.

Pederson E.D., et al (1995)[25] conducted a study to measure five host response indicators namely α-2 macroglobulin, α-1 antitrypsin, C-reactive protein, cathepsin G and elastase by enzyme linked immunosorbent assays on unstimulated whole saliva samples from 45 adults. They examined 5 group representing oral health (I), gingivitis II, moderate periodontitis (III), severe periodontitis (IV) and edentulous volunteers (V). The levels of host-response indicators for group I were significantly lower. Group I – IV showed significant increase in a positive monotonic manner. The findings demonstrate that except for α1- antitrypsin, their levels were directly related to an individuals periodontal status.

Sibraa P.D., et al (1991)[26] conducted a study to evaluate direct and indirect immunodot techniques as to their potential in easily quantifying acute phase proteins within periodontally diseased and healthy site GCF. Indirect immunodots (GCF eluates dotted onto nitrocellulose membrane) using monoclonal antibodies and a radio active isotope label were used to identify and establish relative amounts of CRP and α-2 macroglobulin (A2M) in 2 diseased and 2 healthy sites in 24 periodontitis patients. Periodontally lower concentrations of A2M than healthy sites, but CRP levels did not vary significantly between healthy and diseased sites.

Norman M.E., et al (1979)[27] conducted a study to determine if the early accumulation of plaque in experimental gingivitis is associated with systemic alterations in acute phase serum proteins, Ig and complement. Serial serum specimens were obtained from experimental subjects and matched controls. The data suggested that subtle degrees of systemic complement activation occur in experimental gingivitis, but are only detected by sensitive functional assays.

CRP AND CARDIOVASCULAR

CRP is an extremely sensitive, non-specific, acute phase reactant produced in response to most forms of tissue injury, infection and inflammation and regulated by cytokines, including IL-1, 6 and TNF-α. Circulating CRP is exclusively produced by hepatocytes. They may arise in the atheromatous lesions themselves and reflect the extent of atherosclerosis and the local inflammation that predisposes to plaque instability, rupture and occlusive thrombosis. On the other hand, increased CRP production may result from inflammation elsewhere in the body that is somehow proatherogenic and procoagulant chronic low-grade infections may be associated with increased risk of CHD, as in the chronic inflammation of rheumatoid arthritis. Many coagulation proteins, including fibrinogen, are acute phase reactants; elevation of fibrinogen is a well recognized risk factor for coronary events and increased CRP values may just be a signal of acute phase response in general.[28]

However, there is substantial evidence that CRP may contribute directly to the pathogenesis of atherothrombosis. CRP is a ligand binding protein that binds to the plasma membranes of damaged cells. Aggregated but not soluble native CRP selectively binds LDL and VLDL from whole plasma and could thereby participate in their atherogenic accumulation. Complexed CRP also activates complement and can be pro-inflammatory whereas CRP has recently been found to be a potent stimulator of tissue factor production by macrophages in vitro. Tissue factor is the main initiator of coagulation in vivo, and its local concentration in the arterial wall is clearly related to coronary thrombotic events. There are conflicting reports about the presence of CRP in atheromatous lesions, and claims that CRP affects platelet function are also controversial. However, the capacity of CRP to enhance tissue factor production suggests of possible causative link between increased CRP values and coronary events.[28]

It has recently been demonstrated that anti-inflammatory agents such as aspirin reduced the risk of acute coronary events related to high levels of CRP.[29]

Doo Y.C., et al (2001)[30] conducted a study on 150 patients with a diagnosis of unstable angina. The inclusion criterion was angina at rest, within 48 hrs before admission. Patients with concomitant inflammatory disease, cancer, known thrombotic disorders, vascular heart disease and major surgery or trauma within the previous month were excluded. Blood samples were taken at baseline, 24 and 48 hrs and assessed for serum CRP and IL-6. Blood samples for creatine kinase (CK) and troponin-T measurements were also drawn at admission and at 24 hrs after admission coronary angiography was performed in all patients. They observed that elevated levels of CRP are relatively common and that β-blockers may play a role in decreasing the levels of IL-6 and CRP in patients with unstable angina.

Chew, et al (2001)[31] showed that elevated baseline CRP levels before percutaneous coronary intervention (PCI) are associated with a progressive increase in the risk of death or myocardial infarction at 30 days. The independent association of risk attributable to the marker CRP remained, even after adjusting for a number of baseline variables that are known to influence early events after PCI.

Hashimoto H., et al (2001)[32] conducted a study to evaluate the role of an elevated plasma concentration of high sensitivity CRP

(Hs(CRP) as a strong predictor of cardiovascular events. The study included 179 outpatients 40 to 79 years of age who were treated for traditional risk factors for cardiovascular disease. The patients had no evidence of advanced carotid atherosclerosis at the time of baseline examination. Patients underwent repeated ultrasonographic evaluation of the carotid arteries for 35 ± 10 months. Blood samples were collected for hs-CRP measurements. Based on focal intima-media thickening ≥ 1.1mm representing plaque, plaque number and plaque score were calculated. They concluded that during the early stages of carotid atherosclerosis, the hsCRP concentration is a marker of carotid atherosclerotic activity rather than the extent of atherosclerosis.

Ridker P.M., Stampfer M.J. and Rifai N. (2001)[33] conducted a study to compare the predictive value of 11 lipid and nonlipid biomarkers as risk factors for development of symptomatic peripheral arterial disease (PAD). Plasma samples were collected at baseline from 14916 initially healthy US male physicians aged 40 to 84 yrs, of whom 140 subsequently developed symptomatic PAD cases ; 140 age and smoking status matched men who remained free of vascular disease during an average 9 year follow-up period were randomly selected as controls. Incident PAD, as determined by baseline total cholesterol, HDL-C, LDL-C, total cholesterol–HDL-C ratio, triglycerides, homocysteine, CRP, lipoprotein (a), fibrinogen and apolipoproteins (apo) A-1 and B-100. They concluded that out of 11 atherothrombotic biomarkers assessed at baseline, the total cholesterol–HDL-C ratio and CRP were the strongest independent predictors of development of peripheral arterial disease. CRP

29

provided additive prognostic information over standard lipid measures.

Ridker P.M. (2001)[34] stated that inflammation plays a major role in atherothrombosis and measurement of inflammatory markers such as hsCRP may provide a novel method for detecting individuals at high risk of plaque rupture. Several large-scale prospective studies demonstrate that hsCRP is a strong independent predictor of future myocardial infarction and stroke among apparently healthy men and women. Recent data describing CRP within atheromatous plaque, as a correlate of endothelial dysfunction, and as having a direct role in cell adhesion molecular expression raise the possibility that CRP may also be a potential target for therapy and play an important role as an adjunct for global risk assessment in primary prevention of cardiovascular disease.

Koji Yasojima, et al (2001)[35] conducted a study to evaluate the role of CRP and complement as major mediators of inflammation in atherosclerotic plaques. They used reverse transcriptase-polymerase chain reaction technique to detect the mRNA's for CRP and the classical complement components of C_1 to C_9 in both normal arterial and plaque tissue, establishing that they can be endogenously generated by arteries. They compared that CRP mRNA levels of plaque levels were 10.2 fold higher than normal artery and 7.2 fold higher than liver. They showed by Western blotting that, the proteins levels of CRP and complement proteins were also up-regulated in plaque tissue and that there was full activation of the classical complement pathway. By in situ hybridization, they detected that intense signals for CRP and C_4

mRNA's in smooth muscle like cells and macrophages in the thickened intima of plaque. By immunohistochemistry they showed co-localization of CRP and the membrane attach complex of complement. They showed macrophage infiltration of plaque tissue by immunohistochemistry. They also detected up-regulation in plaque tissue of mRNA's for the macrophage markers CD11b and HLA-DR as well as their protein products. Because CRP is a complement activator and activated complement attacks cells in plaque tissue, they provided evidence of a self-sustaining autotoxin mechanism operating within the plaques as a precursors to thrombotic events.

Ridker P.M., et al (2000)[36] conducted a study to assess the role of inflammation in the pathogenesis of cardiovascular events and measured the markers of inflammation that had been proposed as risk factors. 28,263 apparently healthy post menopausal women were followed for a 3yr period. The markers included hsCRP, serum amyloid A, IL-6 and soluble intercellular adhesion molecule type 1 (sICAM-1). Homocysteine, lipids and lipoprotein measurement were also done. Results showed that of the 12 markers measured, hsCRP was the strongest univariate predictor of the risk of cardiovascular events. They concluded that the addition of the measurement of CRP to screening based on lipid levels may provide an improved method of identifying persons at risk for cardiovascular events.

Morrow D.A. and Ridker P.M. (2000)[37] based on observation epidemiologic data documented a positive association between hsCRP and prevalence of coronary artery disease (CAD). Data also documented associations between mild elevation of hsCRP and cardiovascular risk among those without clinical vascular disease as well as those for whom the focus is on secondary prevention. In addition, data have revealed interactions between baseline concentration of hsCRP and the efficacy of common pharmacologic therapies in primary and secondary prevention, suggesting not only that it may be possible to modify the increased risk associated with elevated hsCRP, but also that inflammatory markers may be useful in targeting preventive therapies.

Lagrand W.K., et al (1999)[38] discussed explanations for the associations between CRP and cardiovascular disease. CRP levels within the upper quartile / quintile of the normal range constitute an increased risk for cardiovascular events, both in apparently healthy persons and in persons with pre-existing angina pectoris. High CRP responses after acute myocardial infarction indicate an unfavorable outcome, even after correction for other risk factors. This link between CRP and cardiovascular disease has been considered to reflect the response of the body to the inflammatory reactions in the atherosclerotic (coronary) vessels and adjacent myocardium. However, because CRP localizes in infarcted myocardium (with localization of activated complement), they hypothesized that CRP may directly interact with atherosclerotic vessels or ischemic myocardium by activation of the complement system, merely promoting inflammation and thrombosis. They concluded that CRP constitutes an independent cardiovascular risk factor.

Abdelmouttaleb I., et al (1999)[29] conducted a study to assess the levels of CRP and other risk factors in patients with angiographically documented coronary artery disease compared with healthy volunteers and patients undergoing coronary angiography who had normal coronary angiograms. Ultrasensitive immuno-assay was used to measure CRP levels in 142 patients with coronary disease (Gp 1), 37 patients with normal coronary angiograms (Gp 2), and 37 control healthy subjects (Gp 3). They found a higher level of CRP among Gp1 when compared to Gp2 and Gp3. Furthermore, CRP levels were positively correlated to plasma fibrinogen but not to chlamydia pneumoniae or helicobacter pylori serology. The results of this study suggest that CRP has a strong association with acute coronary events but do not support the hypothesis that CRP is a potent determinant of chronic stable coronary disease.

Wolfgang Koenig M.D., et al (1999)[28] conducted a study using sensitive immunoradiometric assay to examine the association of serum CRP with the incidence of first major coronary heart disease (CHD) event in 936 men 45 to 64 years of age. The subjects, who were sampled at random from the general population, participated in the first MONICA (Monitoring Trends and Determinants in cardiovascular disease) Augsburg survey (1984 to 1985) and were followed for 8 years. Non-fasting blood samples were taken from all subjects at baseline and stored at -70^0C. Serum CRP concentration were measured in a sensitive immunoradiometric assay with monospecific polyclonal and monoclonal antibodies produced by immunization with highly purified CRP. Total and HDL cholesterol levels were measured by enzymatic methods. The result of this study confirm the prognostic relevance of CRP, a sensitive marker of inflammation, to the risk of CHD in a large, randomly selected cohort of initially healthy middle-aged men. They suggest that low-grade inflammation is involved in pathogenesis of atherosclerosis, especially its thromboocclusive complications.

Haverkate F., et al (1997)[39] conducted a study to investigate the existence and possible significance of the acute phase responses of CRP and another sensitive reactant, serum amyloid A protein (SAA), in patients with unstable or stable angina. Ultra-sensitive immunoassays were used to measure CRP and SAA concentration in plasma from 2121 patients with angina (stable, unstable, atypical). The results were as follows : concentration of CRP at study entry were associated with coronary events in patients with stable or unstable angina: there was about a 2 fold increase in the risk of a coronary event in patients whose CRP concentration was in the 5th quintile (> 3.6mg/L), compared with the 1st four quintiles. CRP concentration were positively correlated with age, smoking, body mass index, triglycerides, extent of coronary stenosis, history of MI and lower ejection fraction. By contrast, concentration of SAA were not associated with risk of a coronary event. They concluded that raised circulating concentrations of CRP are predictors of coronary events in patients with stable or unstable angina.

Mendall M.A., et al (1996)[40] conducted a study to test the hypothesis that minor chronic insults such as smoking, chronic bronchitis and two persistent bacterial infections may be associated with increases in CRP concentration within the normal range and that variations in the CRP concentration in turn may be associated with levels of cardiovascular risk factors and chronic coronary heart disease. A random sample of 388 men aged 50-69 years were examined. Measurements of serum CRP concentration was done by in house enzyme linked immuosorbent assay (ELISA) and coronary heart disease by the Rose Angina questionnaire and Minnesota coded electrocardiograms. The results of their study showed that an increasing age, smoking, symptoms of chronic bronchitis, Helicobacter pylori and chlamydia pneumoniae infections and body mass index were all associated with raised concentrations of CRP. CRP concentration was associated with raised serum fibrinogen, sialic acid, total cholesterol, triglycerides, glucose and apolipoprotein B values. CRP concentration was negatively associated with high density lipoprotein cholesterol concentration. CRP concentration was also strongly associated with coronary heart disease. They concluded that body's response to inflammation may play an important part in influencing the progression of atherosclerosis.

CRP AND RHEUMATOID ARTHRITIS

Several studies have demonstrated a correlation between elevated serum acute-phase proteins and the magnitude of joint destruction in rheumatoid arthritis. Evidence is also available suggesting that CRP levels provide a sensitive and objective indicator of disease activity and clearly reflect the response to therapy of rheumatoid arthritis. In rheumatoid arthritis patient plasma IL-10 increased and IL-6 and CRP were significantly elevated versus controls. CRP levels were highly correlated with plasma IL-6 in patients with other inflammatory arthritides, particularly psoriatic and HLAB27-positive spondyloarthritis.[9]

Suppression of elevated CRP in patients with active rheumatoid arthritis is associated with improvement in functional score where as persistent elevation in CRP is associated with functional determination. CRP values correlated closely with radiological progression of joint disease in rheumatoid arthritis. The CRP accurately predicted outcome from 6months after presentation and may be used in a decision support system.[13]

Mercado F.B., et al (2001)[41] conducted a study to study a population of rheumatoid arthritis patients and determine the extent of their periodontal disease and correlate this with various indicators of rheumatoid arthritis.65 consecutive patients were examined for periodontitis and rheumatoid arthritis (RA). Specific measures for periodontitis included probing depths, attachment loss, bleeding scores, plaque scores, and radiographic bone loss scores. Measures of RA included tender joint analysis, swollen joint analysis, pain index, physician's global assessment on a visual analogue scale, health assessment questionnaire, levels of CRP and ESR rate. They found that levels of CRP and ESR were the principal parameters which could be associated with periodontal bone loss. The results of this study provided an evidence of a significant association between periodontitis and rheumatoid arthritis.

Laiho K., et al (2001)[42] conducted a study to evaluate serum CRP concentration in patients with rheumatoid arthritis (RA) undergoing total hip arthroplasty (THA) or total knee arthroplasty (TKA) to ascertain the post operative CRP response. 37consecutive patients who had undergone THA or TKA were included. The CRP concentration was measured in every patient once pre-operatively and every other day for one week post-operatively. They concluded that a rapid rise in the post-operative CRP concentration is normal in patients with RA treated by THA or TKA. The concentration of CRP decreases to the preoperative value in about one week. When the post operative CRP concentration remains raised for several days compared with the pre-operative value or even rises, it may indicate the presence of a complication in those patients.

Cantini F., et al (2000)[43] conducted a study to determine the frequency and clinical features of patients with polymyalgia rheumatica (PMR) and normal erythrocyte sedimentation rate (ESR at diagnosis or during relapse / recurrence and to evaluate the usefulness of CRP and ESR in the assessment of PMR activity. At diagnosis and during follow up, ESR (Westergren method) and CRP (nephelometry) were measured in 177consecutive patients. They found that patients with normal ESR were predominantly men and had lower CRP levels, systemic signs and symptoms were more frequent in patients with higher ESR. CRP was high in 62% of episodes of relapse/ recurrence. They concluded that PMR with a normal ESR at diagnosis was infrequent and ESR was a superior predictor of relapse than CRP. However, CRP was a more sensitive indicator of current disease activity.

Plant M.J., et al (2000)[44] conducted a study to investigate the hypothesis that when there is suppression of disease activity as judged by the CRP level, new joint involvement is reduced to a greater extent than is progression in already damaged joints. 359 patients were studied as part of a 5year randomized, prospective, open-label study of disease – modifying anti-rheumatic drug therapy. Time averaged CRP was calculated from samples obtained every 6 months and patients were divided into groups with CRP values of < 6, 6 - < 12, 12- < 25 and > or = 25mg/L. Radiographs of the hands and feet were scored by the Larsen method; a damaged joint was defined as one with a score of > or = 2. They concluded that high CRP levels over time are associated with greater radiologic progression.

Dougados M., et al (1999)[45] conducted a study to evaluate CRP as a potential useful criteria of symptomatic severity of ankylosing spondilitis (AS) in 443 patients with axial involvement. During the 6 weeks of the study, patients received either a placebo or an active non-steroidal anti-inflammatory drug (NSAID). It was found that at baseline, CRP was increased in 173 patients. They concluded that night pain and laboratory signs of inflammation were the most significant variables explaining the changes in CRP values. The capacity of CRP to discriminate between an active NSAID and a placebo was found to be moderate. This study suggested that an increase in CRP in patients with AS with axial involvement is not a rare phenomenon and might be correlated with the clinical severity of the disease.

Conrozier T., et al (1998)[46] conducted a study to compare serum CRP levels measured using a highly sensitive immunonephelometry method in patients with rapidly destructive versus slowly progressive hip osteoarthritis. Ten patients meeting criteria for rapidly destructive hip osteoarthritis were compared to 25 patients with slowly progressive hip osteoarthritis defined as less than 0.20 mm joint space loss over the last year. The detection threshold for CRP was 0.17 mg/L. They concluded that rapidly destructive hip osteoarthritis may be associated with some degree of inflammation reflected by a small but significant increase in serum CRP levels.

Youinou P., et al (1990)[47] conducted a study to evaluate the CRP response in rheumatoid arthritis patients with secondary Sjogren's syndrome. They found the levels of serum CRP significantly higher in the presence than in the absence of secondary Sjogren's syndrome in patients with rheumatoid arthritis, while the values of ESR and serum fibrinogen were not significantly different. They found the levels of CRP normal in 22 out of 24 patients with primary Sjogren's syndrome.

STATINS AND CRP

The acute phase response is activated by ongoing intra arterial inflammation. Resident macrophages, stimulated by oxidized LDL (cholesterol and phospholipid) or other agonists, secrete pro-inflammatory cytokines and expresses tissue factor, thus initiating local inflammation and promoting thrombosis. IL-6, the principal cytokine that induces the acute-phase response, can be found in atheromatous coronary arteries in the patient with unstable angina, the condition in which intra-arterial inflammation has been implicated most convincingly. The blood CRP levels have not correlated with the extent of coronary artery disease observable on angiography in patients with angina, however, raising doubts that intracoronary inflammation alone can account for the observed elevations in CRP levels; inflammation in other vessels could obviously contribute as might intravascular infection, if it exists. Statin drugs, which inhibit hydroxymethyl glutaryl co-enzyme A reductase, would prevent atherosclerosis and inhibit the acute phase response by diminishing the deposition of LDL particles rich in cholesterol and phospholipids (arachidonate) in macrophages and smooth muscle cells in the arterial wall.[48]

Recent studies suggest that statin therapy may also prevent diabetes mellitus, osteoporosis and Alzheimer's disease. In each of these conditions, as in coronary disease, the beneficial effect of the drugs might be attributed to their LDL-lowering activities, their anti-inflammatory activities or both. If statins inhibit the acute-phase response by diminishing the intravascular deposition of cholesterol and phospholipids, more potent statin treatment will probably not interfere with acute phase responses to infection, injury and other types of stress. If they broadly inhibit the acute-phase response, on the other hand, the ultimate preventive effect of these remarkable drugs could be limited, at least in part, by their ability to attempt the beneficial function of that response.[48]

Feldman M., et al (2001)[49] conducted a study to evaluate the effect of low dose aspirin on serum CRP levels. Elevated circulating concentration of CRP, an inflammatory marker, increase the risk of thrombotic cardiovascular diseases such as myocardial infarction(MI). Moreover, low-dose aspirin therapy has been reported to be more effective in preventing MI in men with higher CRP levels than it is in those with lower levels, raising the possibility that aspirin prevents thrombosis by reducing vascular inflammation. Effects of aspirin on serum CRP were studied. Results of this study showed no significant changes in serum CRP levels from baseline with daily low dose aspirin regimens or with placebo treatment. They concluded that low doses of aspirin markedly inhibit platelet COX-1 activity, as manifested by a profound decline in platelet derived serum Tx B_2 concentration, have no detectable effect on serum CRP levels in healthy men and women.

Ridker P.M., et al (2001)[50] hypothesized that statins might prevent coronary events in persons with elevated CRP levels who did not have overt hyperlipidemia. They measured levels of CRP at base line and after one year in 5742 participants in a 5 yr randomized trial of lovastatin for the primary prevention of acute coronary events. The results of this study showed that the rate of coronary events increased significantly with increases in the base-line levels of CRP. Lovastatin therapy reduced the CRP level by 14.8%. They concluded that statin therapy may be effective in the primary prevention of coronary events among subjects with relatively low lipid levels but with elevated CRP level.

Ridker P.M, Rifai N. and Lowenthal S.P. (2001)[51] conducted a study to show that long term therapy with hydroxymethyl glutaryl coenzyme A reductase inhibitors (statins) reduce levels of CRP. They measured CRP, LDL and HDL cholesterol among 785 patients with primary hypercholesterolemia at baseline and after 8 weeks of therapy with either 0.4 or 0.8mg of cerivastatin. Overall, cerivastatin resulted in a 13.3% reduction in median CRP levels and a 24.5% reduction in mean CRP levels. They concluded that, CRP levels were significantly reduced within 8 weeks of initiating cerivastatin therapy in a lipid-independent manner.

Eisenberg M.S., et al (2000)[52] hypothesized that plasma levels of CRP and IL-6, markers for systemic inflammation, would correlate with cardiac transplant graft survival. They studied 99 consecutive cardiac transplant recipients. Plasma levels of CRP and IL-6 were measured by their respective ELISA. Patients were divided into 2 groups : those who died or required retransplantation and those who survived without the need for retransplantation. It was observed that although IL-6 did not relate to graft failure, CRP level was predictive of allograft failure. They concluded that elevated plasma levels of CRP are associated with subsequent allograft failure in cardiac transplant recipients.

Strandberg T.E., Vanhanen H. and Tikkanen M.J. (2000)[53] conducted a study on 60 hypercholesterolaemic coronary patients. It was observed that hypolipidaemic 3 hydroxy-3methyl glutaryl coenzyme A (HMG-CoA) reductase inhibitor (statin) treatment reduces cardiac risk and CRP concentration. Serum lipids and CRP were measured before treatment at baseline and after 12 months of statin treatment. The following conclusions were drawn ; LDL cholesterol was substantially decreased and HDL cholesterol increased during statin treatment. CRP decreased significantly during treatment, and the changes of CRP were significantly associated with changes in LDL cholesterol or triglycerides.

Horne B.D., et al (2000)[54] conducted a study to evaluate the joint predictive value of lipid and CRP levels, as well as a possible interaction between statin therapy and CRP, for survival after angiographic diagnosis of coronary artery disease (CAD). Blood samples were collected from 985 patients diagnosed angiographically with severe CAD (stenosis) and tested for total cholesterol (TC), LDL, HDL and CRP levels. Key risk factors including initiation of statin therapy, were recorded and subjects were followed for an average of 3 yrs. They concluded that lipid levels drawn at angiography were not predictive of survival in this population, but initiation of statin therapy was associated with improved survival regardless of the lipid levels. The benefit of statin therapy occurred primarily in patients with elevated CRP.

Ridker P.M., et al (1999)[55] conducted a study to evaluate whether long term therapy with pravastatin, an agent that reduces cardiovascular risk, might alter levels of CRP, an inflammatory parameter. The CRP levels were measured at baseline and at 5yrs in 472 randomly selected patients who remained free of recurrent coronary events during follow up. They concluded that among survivors of myocardial infarction on standard therapy plus placebo, CRP levels tended to increase over 5yrs of follow up. In contrast, randomization to pravastatin resulted in significant reductions in this inflammatory marker that were not related to the magnitude of lipid alterations observed.

CRP AND OTHER DISEASES

Pradhan A.D., et al (2001)[13] in a study concluded that elevated levels of CRP and IL-6 predict the development of type 2 Diabetes mellitus. These data support a possible role for inflammation in diabetogenesis.

Kawai T., (2000)[25] stated that acute phase proteins are synthesized mainly in the liver cells, induced by various inflammatory cytokines which are produced by activated macrophages / monocytes at the inflammatory sites. CRP is a principal acute phase protein, and increased most significantly upon various inflammation.

False negative results may be recognized in the patients with viral infections, collagen diseases such as systemic lupus erythematosus, dermatomyositis, ulcerative colitis, Sjogrens syndrome, leukemia, cerebral infarction etc.

Tatara R. and Imai H. (2000)[57] found that diagnostic accuracy of a single CRP determination was equivalent to that of the most effective combination test. They found that patients with meningitis in whom serum CRP values are determined at least 12 h after the onset of fever and are < 2 mg /dl are far less likely to have bacterial meningitis.

Dougados M., et al (1999)[45] in a study suggested that an increase in CRP in ankylosing spondylitis patients with axial involvement is not a rare phenomenon and might be correlated with the clinical severity of the disease.

Visser M., et al (1999)[58] in a study showed that higher BMI is associated with higher CRP concentration, even among young adults aged 17 to 39 years. These findings suggest a state of low-grade systemic inflammation in overweight and obese persons.

Bakri H.A., et al (1998)[59] in a study concluded that mixed connective tissue disease patients have high immunoglobulin levels as well as high CRP levels and that this situation is compatible with the observed increase in both type I and type II cytokine levels.

Materials Provided With CRP Latex Kit :

Box –1 contains reagents :

1) CRP latex reagent 1vial.
2) CRP positive control 1 vial.
3) CRP negative control 1 vial.

Box –2 contains accessories :

1) Disposable sample droppers 25 nos.
2) Disposable mixing sticks 25 nos.
3) Test slide 1 no.
4) Product insert 1 no.

Testing Procedure :

The detection of CRP was performed by "Latex slide agglutination method".

Procedural Precautions Undertaken :

1) Only unhaemolysed, non lipemic and non turbid serum sample was used for greater accuracy.
2) All reagents and the test samples were brought to room temperature before use.
3) A new plastic dropper and mixing stick for each sample was used.
4) The test slide was neatly cleaned before use for each sample.

Test Procedure (For Qualitative Measurement) :

1) Pipette one drop of test sample on to the identified ring of the test slide using a disposable dropper provided along with the kit.

45

2) Mix latex reagent by gentle shaking of the vial. Add one drop of CRP latex reagent to the drop of test sample added on circle of test slide.

3) Thoroughly mix the each sample with Latex reagent using separate mixing stick uniformly within the full area of the circle of test slide.

4) Slowly rock the slide exactly for two minutes and observe for agglutination under a high intensity light source.

Test Procedure (For Semiquantitative Measurement) :

1) Prepare serial dilution of the test sample (1:2, 1:4, 1:8) to be titered, using 0.9% NaCl solution (saline) in neat and clean labeled test tubes.

2) Pipette the diluted sample from each tube onto the identified circle of test slide.

3) Add one drop of CRP latex reagent to the circle containing diluted sample and mix well using mixing stick.

4) Slowly rock the slide exactly for two minutes and observe for agglutination under a high intensity light source.

Result Interpretation :

Qualitative Method :

Visible agglutination is a positive test result and indicates the presence of detectable level of CRP in test specimen.

No agglutination is a negative test result and indicates the absence of detectable level of CRP in test specimen.

Semi Quantitative Method :

The highest dilution of the test sample showing agglutination corresponds to the amount of CRP (mg/dl) present in the test sample.

The concentration of CRP can be calculated as follows :

CRP (mg/dl) in test specimen = factor of 0.6 x Δ^*

Δ^* = highest dilution of serum showing agglutination.

DISCUSSION

C-reactive protein (CRP) is an acute-phase reactant produced by the liver in response to diverse inflammatory stimuli, including heat, trauma, infection and hypoxia (Pepys M.B. and Baltz. 1983).[19] In patients with overwhelming systemic infection, serum levels of CRP can exceed 100mg/L, providing a useful marker for tracking the course of the infection. However, the clinical relevance of much smaller increases in CRP has been highlighted recently in epidemiological studies demonstrating that individuals with "high-normal" values of CRP have increased risk for chronic diseases that have an inflammatory basis, including cardiovascular disease.[19]

Established risk factors for "high-normal" values of CRP within the general population include older age, cigarette smoking, chronic bacterial infections and chronic bronchial inflammation (Palosuo, et al 1986, Saikku, et al 1992, Patel, et al 1995, Mendall M.A., et al 1996, Ridker P.M., et al 1997). However raised CRP levels have been observed among individuals with no apparent established risk factors for elevated CRP, suggesting that other pathological conditions may constitute an additional stimulus for a systemic inflammatory response among some individuals.[19]

CRP is an abnormal protein that appears in the blood in acute stages of various inflammatory disorders, but is undetectable in the blood of healthy individuals. CRP is a serum protein which is synthesized in the liver only during an inflammatory disease. It is normally present as a trace constituent of plasma (0 to 0.6 mg/dl).[3]

Mustard R. A., (1987)[3] explained that serum CRP concentration increases within 12 hours and reaches peak levels within 24 to 48 hours. The serum half-life of CRP is less than 24

49

hours. CRP values shows peak levels within 1 to 3 days of the acute stimulus and fall rapidly with cessation of the inflammatory reaction.[41]

An elevated serum concentration of CRP is evidence of an active tissue – damaging process and CRP measurement thus provides a simple screening test for organic disease and inflammatory diseases. Increased CRP production is a very early and sensitive response to most forms of microbial infections. It is an index of disease activity and response to therapy in some inflammatory, infective and ischaemic conditions. The test is not specific, since CRP appears in blood as a response to various other inflammatory conditions also.[1]

This CRP production by hepatocytes occurs at the expense of albumin and other constitutive proteins, a process labeled "reprioritization" of hepatic protein synthesis. However, competing demands for protein synthesis in case of acute, overwhelming inflammation can lead to anomalous short term changes in acute – phase reactants. While these short-term discrepancies may be important considerations in the monitoring of temporal changes in acute phase response to major trauma, it seems unlikely that they would be sufficient to bias the current cross-sectional associations between periodontal disease and high-normal CRP levels.[19]

Periodontal disease is a chronic inflammatory process that occurs in response to a predominantly gram-negative bacterial infection originating from dental plaque. While the etiological role of bacteria has been firmly established in vitro and in vivo, it is only recently that researchers have begun to identify local and systemic inflammatory processes that encourage a pathological response to an initial, commensal microflora (Page R.C. 1995, Offenbacher S. 1996). Equally compelling is the evidence from experimental studies demonstrating enhanced release of inflammatory mediators (for eg; PGE_2, IL-1β, TNF-α) from peripheral monocytes drawn from patients with periodontal disease when those monocytes are challenged, in vitro, with bacterial lipopolysaccharide (Shapira, et al 1994, Salvi, et al 1997).[22] These cytokines are involved in destruction of both periodontal connective tissue and alveolar bone. They also initiate a systemic acute phase response. Recent studies have shown that C-reactive protein (CRP) serum levels in patients with periodontal disease are elevated.[5]

In case of periodontal disease, the magnitude of the association was comparable with that identified for conditions such as chronic bronchitis and cigarette smoking. The stronger effect of oral status among the group with no established risk factors probably reflects the absence of other contributing causes of an acute-phase response, and in many respects this group provides a more controlled test of the potential for oral conditions to elicit an acute phase response. This modifying effect may further explain why some previous studies examining established risk factors for CRP found raised CRP levels even among "apparently healthy" people (Ridker P.M., et al 1997).[4]

Periodontitis has been proposed as having an etiological or modulating role in cardiovascular and cerebrovascular disease (Matilla, et al 1989, Beck J.D., et al 1996, Wu T., et al 2000), diabetes (Grossi and Genco 1998), respiratory disease (Hayes, et al 1998) and adverse pregnancy outcome. (Offenbacher S., et al 1996).

There is still much debate regarding the nature and degree to which this may happen (Howell, et al 2001).[54]

Several mechanisms have been proposed to explain or support such theories. One of these is based around the potential for the inflammatory phenomenon of periodontitis to have effects by the systemic dissemination of locally produced mediators such as C-reactive protein (CRP), interleukin-1beta (IL-1β) and –6 (IL-6) and tumor necrosis factor-alpha (TNF -α) (Gemmell, et al 1997, Kornman, et al 1997). This concept has been supported by work suggesting that elevated levels of a number of inflammatory molecules may be accurate indicators of cardiovascular risk.[23] Moderate elevation of serum CRP is a risk factor for cardiovascular disease among apparently healthy individuals although factors that create this inflammatory response in absence of systemic illness have not been clarified (Slade G.D., et al 2000).[56]

There is substantial evidence that CRP may contribute directly to the pathogenesis of atherothrombosis. CRP is a ligand binding protein that binds to the plasma membrane of damaged cells. Aggregated but not soluble native CRP selectively binds Low Density Lipoprotein (LDL) and Very Low Density Lipoprotein (VLDL) from whole plasma and could thereby participate in their atherogenic accumulation. Complexed CRP also activates complement and can be proinflammatory whereas CRP has recently been found to be a potent stimulator of tissue factor production by macrophages in vitro. Tissue factor is the main initiator of coagulation in vivo and its local concentration in the arterial wall is clearly related to coronary thrombotic events. However, the capacity of CRP to enhance tissue factor production suggests a possible causative link between increased CRP values and coronary events.[28]

The mechanism by which CRP participates in cardiovascular diseases is not clear; however CRP may activate the complement system and be involved in foam cell formation in atheromas. However other associations of CRP to periodontal infection have not been reported.[5]

Furthermore, it has been proposed that patients with periodontitis may have elevated circulating levels of some of these inflammatory markers (Beck et al 1998, Page 1998) although there are limited published data to support this (Collins, et al 1994, Noack B., et al 2001).[14]

As seen from the above review of available information the serum CRP estimation proved to be a useful and a sensitive diagnostic indicator of inflammatory disorders or active tissue – destroying processes and in monitoring and assessing various inflammatory and infectious conditions and as a guideline to therapy. It was also used in monitoring post-operative complications and in their management.[3]

Consequently, if a relationship exists between periodontal disease and systemic CRP within the population at large, it has the potential for substantial clinical relevance in helping to explain circumstances in which an intra-oral source of infection can create a systemic inflammatory response, therefore placing "apparently healthy" patients at increased risk of cardiovascular disease. Such an association could also represent a mechanism underlying recent epidemiological findings that oral diseases appear to be risk factors for cardiovascular disease (Beck J.D., et al 1996).[4]

BIBLIOGRAPHY

1. Pepys M.B. (1981): C-reactive protein fifty years on. Lancet; 21: 653-56.

2. Gewurz H., et al (1982): C-reactive protein and the acute phase response Adv Intern Med; 27: 345-372.

3. Norman M.E., et al (1979): Studies of host responses during experimental gingivitis in humans. J Periodontol Res; 14(5) : 361-69.

4. Slade G.D., et al (2000): Acute phase inflammatory response to periodontal disease in the US population. J Dent Res; 79: 49-57.

5. Noack B., et al (2001): Periodontal infections contribute to elevated systemic C-reactive protein level. J Periodontol; 72(9) : 1221-27.

6. Tucci A., et al (1983): Biosynthesis and Post-synthetic processing of human CRP. J Immunol; 131(5): 2416-19.

7. Czalai A.J., et al (1999) : CRP : Structural biology and host defence function. Clin – Chem Lab Med; 37(3): 265-70.

8. Thompson D., Pepys M.B. and Wood S.P. (1999): The physiologic structure of human CRP and its complex with phosphocholine. Structure; 7(2): 169-77.

9. Ebersole J.L. and Cappelli D. (2000): Acute phase reactants in infections and inflammatory diseases. Periodontology 2000; 23: 19-49.

10. Mold C., Gewurz H. and Du Clos T.W. (1999): Regulation of complement activation by CRP. Immunopharmacology; 42(1-3): 23-30.

11. Mortensen R.F. and Zhong W. (2000): Regulation of phagocytic leucocyte activities by CRP. J-Leukoc-Biol; 67(4): 495-500.

12. Vetter M.L., et al (1982): Effects of CRP on human lymphocyte responsiveness. J Immunol; 130(5): 2121-26.

13.   Craig R.G., et al (2003) : Relationship of destructive periodontal disease to the acute phase response. J Periodontol; 74(7) : 1007-16.

14. Ide M., et al (2003): Effect of treatment of chronic periodontitis on levels of serum markers of acute-phase inflammatory and vascular responses. J Clin Periodontol ; 30: 334-40.

15. Wu T., et al (2001): Periodontal disease, CRP and ischemic stroke. Arch-Intern Med; 161(9) : 1234-5.

16. Wu T., et al (2000): Examination of the relation between periodontal health status and cardiovascular risk factors: Serum total and high density lipoprotein cholesterol, C-Reactive protein and plasma fibrinogen. Am J Epi; 151: 273-82.

17. Williams R.C. and Offenbacher S. (2000): Periodontal Medicine : the emergency of a new branch of periodontology. Periodontology 2000; 23: 9-12.

18. Loos B.G., et al (2000): Elevation of systemic markers related to cardiovascular diseases in the peripheral blood of periodontitis patients. J Periodontol; 71(10): 1528-34.

19. Slade G.D., et al (2000): Acute phase inflammatory response to periodontal disease in the US population. J Dent Res; 79: 49-57.

20. Ebersole J.L., et al (1999): Systemic manifestations of periodontitis in the non-human primate. J Periodontol Res ; 34: 358-62.

21. Frederiksson M.I., et al (1999): Effect of periodontitis and smoking on blood leucocytes and acute phase proteins. J periodontal ; 70: 1355-60.

22. Glurich I., et al (1998): Inflammation, periodontal disease and Atherogenesis. A possible risk. J Dent Res ; 77 (spec issue): 666 (Abst 277).

23. Ebersole J.L., et al (1997): Systemic acute phase reactants, C-reactive protein and haptoglobin in Adult Periodontitis. Clin Exp Immunol; 107(2): 347-52.

24. Meurman J.H., et al (1997): Oral infections in home living elderly patients admitted to an acute geriatric ward. J Dent Res; 76(6): 1271-6.

25. Pedersen E.D., et al (1995): Salivary levels of α-2 macroglobulin, α-1 antitrypsin, CRP, Cathepsin G and elastase in humans with or without destructive periodontal disease. Arch Oral Biol; 40(12): 1151-5.

26. Sibraa P.D., et al (1991): Acute phase protein detection and quantification in gingival crevicular fluid by direct and indirect immunodot techniques. J Clin Periodontol; 18: 101-6.

27. Norman M.E., et al (1979): Studies of host responses during experimental gingivitis in humans. J Periodontol Res; 14(5) : 361-69.

28. Wolfgang Koenig M.D., et al (1999): CRP, a sensitive marker of inflammation predicts future risk of coronary heart disease in initially healthy middle aged men. Circulation, 19; 99(2): 237-42.

29. Abdelmouttaleb I., et al (1999): CRP and coronary artery disease additional evidence of the implication of an

inflammatory process in acute coronary syndromes. Am Heart J; 137(2) : 346-51.

30. Doo Y.C., et al (2001) : Effect of beta blockers on expression of IL-6 and CRP in patients with unstable angina pectoris. Am J Cardiol, 15; 88(4): 422-4.

31. Chew, et al (2001): CRP: linking inflammation to cardiovascular complications. Circulation; 104(9) : 974-5.

32. Hashimoto H., et al (2001): C-reactive protein is an independent predictor of the rate of increase in early carotid atherosclerosis. Circulation, 3; 104(1) : 63-7.

33. Ridker P.M., Stampfer M.J. and Rifai N. (2001): Novel risk factors for systemic atherosclerosis : a comparison of C-reactive protein, fibrinogen, homocysteine, lipoprotein (a) and standard cholesterol screening as predictors of peripheral arterial disease. J Am Med Assoc, 16; 285 (19): 2481-5.

34. Ridker P.M., et al (2001): High-sensitivity of CRP : potential adjunct for global risk assessment in the primary prevention of cardiovascular disease. Circulation, 3; 103(13): 1813-8.

35. Koji Yasojima, et al (2001): Generation of CRP and complement components in atherosclerotic plaques. J Pathology ; 58(3): 1039-51.

36. Ridker P.M., et al (2000): C-reactive protein and other markers of inflammation in the prediction of cardiovascular disease in women. N Engl J Med; 342: 836-43.

37. Morrow D.A. and Ridker P.M. (2000): C-reactive protein, inflammation and coronary risk. Med Clin North Am; 84(1): 149-61,ix.

38. Lagrand W.K., et al (1999): C-reactive protein as a cardiovascular risk factor: more than an epiphenomenon. Circulation, 6; 100(1): 96-102.

39. Haverkate F., et al (1997): Production of C-Reactive protein and risk of coronary events in stable and unstable angina. European concerted action on thrombosis and disabilities angina pectoris study group. Lancet; 349: 462-66.

40. Mendall M.A., et al (1996): C-reactive protein and its relation to cardiovascular risk factors a population based cross-sectional study. Br Med J; 312:1061-65.

41. Mercado F.B., et al (2001): Relationship between rheumatoid arthritis and periodontitis. J Periodontol; 72(6): 779-87.

42. Laiho K., et al (2001): Rise in serum CRP after hip and knee arthroplasties in patients with rheumatoid arthritis. Ann-Rheum-Dis; 60(3) : 275-7.

43. Cantini F., et al (2000): ESR and CRP in the evaluation of disease activity and severity in polymyalgia rheumatica: a prospective follow-up study. Semin-Arthritis-Rheum; (1): 17-24.

44. Plant M.J., et al (2000): Relationship between time integrated CRP levels and radiologic progression in patients with rheumatoid arthritis. Arthritis-Rheum; 43(7): 1473-7.

45. Dougadas M., et al (1999) : Clinical relevance of CRP in axial involvement of ankylosing spondylitis. J Rheumatol; 26(4) : 971-4.

46. Conrozier T., et al (1998) : Increased serum C-reactive protein levels by immunonephelometry in patients with rapidly destructive hip osteoarthritis. Rev-Rheum-Engl-Ed; 65(12): 759-65.

47. Youinou P., et al (1990): Raised C-reactive protein response in reheumatoid arthritis patients with secondary Sjogren's syndrome. Rheumatol Int; 10(1): 39-41.

48. Munford R.S. (2001): Statins and the acute phase response. N Engl J Med, 28; 344 (26): 2016-18.

49. Feldman M., et al (2001): Effects of low dose aspirin on serum C-reactive protein levels. J Am Coll Cardiol, 15; 37 (8): 2036-41.

50. Ridker P.M., et al (2001): Measurement of CRP for the targetting of statin therapy in the primary prevention of acute coronary events. N Engl J Med; 344(26): 1959-65.

51. Ridker P.M., Rifai N. and Lowenthal S.P. (2001): Rapid reduction of C-reactive protein with cerivastatin in patients with hypercholesterolemia. Circulation; 103(9): 1191-3.

52. Eisenbeg M.S., et al (2000): Elevated levels of plasma CRP are associated with decreased graft survival in cardiac transplant recipient. Circulation, 24; 102(17) : 2100-4.

53. Strandberg T.E., Vanhanen H. and Tikkanen M.J., (2000): Associations between change in C-reactive protein and serum lipids during statin treatment. Ann Med; 32(8): 579-83.

54. Horne B.D., et al (2000): Divergent effects of hormone therapy on serum markers of inflammation in post menopausal women with coronary artery disease on appropriate medical management. J Am Coll Cardiol, 15; 36 (6) : 1774-80.

55. Ridker P.M., et al (1999): Long-term effects of pravastatin on plasma concentration of C-reactive protein. Circulation; 100: 230-35.

56. Kawai T. (2000): Inflammatory markers, especially the mechanism of increased C-reactive protein. Rinsho-Byori ; 48(8) : 719-21.

57. Tatara R. and Imai H. (2000): Serum C-reactive protein in the differential diagnosis of childhood meningitis. Pediatr Int; 42(5): 541-6.

58. Visser M., et al (1999) : Elevated CRP levels in overweight and obese adults. J Am Med Assoc; 282(22): 2131-5.

59.   Bakri H.A., et al (1998): Increased serum levels of immunoglobulin, CRP, type I and type II cytokines in patients with mixed connective tissue disease. J Auto immun; 11(5) : 503-8.

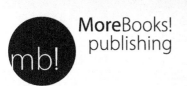
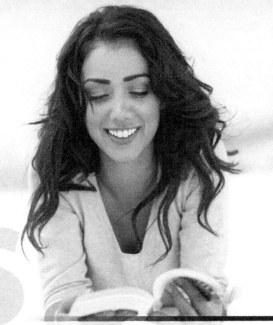

Printed in Great Britain
by Amazon

84101216R00047